HOW TO DO A COMPLETE NATURAL DETOXIFICATION

REMOVE TOXINS FROM YOUR LIVER, DETOXIFY YOUR BODY BEFORE STARTING A DIET, EXPEL TOBACCO FROM YOUR ARTERIES

Jessy M. Brown

Table of Contents

Introduction The Detox Diet

Detoxification occurs daily in our bodies

Our internal organs, the colon, liver, and intestines, help our bodies remove toxic and harmful matter from our bloodstream and tissues. Our systems are often overloaded with waste.

The same air we breathe, and all its pollutants, accumulate in our bodies.

Today's overprocessed foods and environmental pollutants can easily overwhelm our delicate systems and cause toxic matter to accumulate in our bodies.

Detox diets are designed to help your body get rid of the buildup of toxic matter and lose weight.

If you feel slow, have frequent colds,

digestive problems, or just don't feel your best, you may have a toxicity problem. A detox diet will help you cleanse harmful matter from your body and lose weight.

A detox diet will help your body by increasing endurance and energy, making the digestive process easier.

It will help increase mental clarity and decrease allergies. Most detox diets do not include rare or unhealthy foods, just fresh, whole-grain foods such as fruits and vegetables. Eat plenty of fresh fruit, except grapefruit. The enzymes in grapefruit interfere with the proper functioning of enzymes in the liver, so they should not be used during detox diets.

Grapefruit should not be consumed during detoxification programs, but are ideal for any other time.

Fresh vegetables are also excellent in the detox diet

The best vegetables to detoxify are broccoli, garlic, artichokes, beets, cauliflower and red and green vegetables. Avoid corn products, as corn often contains allergens. Rice is also acceptable on a detox diet, and beans, nuts, and seeds are also excellent.

Drink plenty of water

You need about 6 to 8 glasses a day to help your body eliminate toxins. A hydrated body helps your body's organs function optimally. Drink plenty of pure, crystal.... clear water as pure as you can.

A Simple Detox Diet Plan

A simple detox diet plan may involve not eating meat for a couple of days. For a more detailed plan, consult a professional about what to eat at each meal during the detox period. Stay away from meats during your detox program.

Using a detox diet plan can help maximize your health, reduce your weight, and help you feel more energetic and rested.

The truth, when it comes to body detoxification done in a clinic or even a spa, is that it will cost you a good deal of money. In fact, a stay in a detoxification clinic can reach up to ten thousand dollars, depending on the methods and treatments used. So instead of spending so much money on a clinic or even a spa, most people prefer home detox as an effective alternative solution that is cheap and also does the job.

Simple home detox means controlling what you eat and drink. Fortunately it is not a very demanding process as there are no medical procedures involved. However, detoxification at home allows the body to cleanse itself and by eating special diets and supplementing them with natural therapies you can experience a number of benefits while there are no side effects to worry about.

Try a detox diet for a few days. You will
be amazed at how light it will feel!

Detoxification Benefits

Seems a little unpleasant when you're detoxing or cleaning up.

Your body shows some signs that you've accumulated toxins. These toxins can affect the physical condition and health of your entire body. There are times when you feel lazy and stressed. Your body may experience continued pain, diarrhea, constipation, and a feeling of clumsiness. Rapid weight gain and the inability to lose excess weight can also be signs of toxins in the body.

In addition, toxins found in the body are found and stored in fat cells. For Americans who are eating the usual American diet, one person can eventually consume 70 trillion trash cans per cell! When detoxifying your body and cleaning unwanted waste from your cells, you should pay attention to your elimination organs.

There are particular organs in your body that handle cellular waste.

These organs play an important role in the detoxification process for a healthy and fit body.

1) Your liver is the organ that recycles unwanted chemicals in the body. It classifies toxins and sends them to the appropriate organ for elimination during the circulation process. The major elimination organs will support the liver so that these toxins are stored and then eliminated.

2) Lymph glands also play an important role in the elimination of toxins. A network of tubes removes excess waste from the body's cells and carries it to the final disposal organs. The appendix, thymus, tonsils, and spleen are the main lymph glands that assist the body's major organs in cleansing and detoxification.

3) The kidneys help manage the body's water. They maintain the good chemistry of alkaline blood by removing dissolved acid residues. You can help your kidneys work very well by drinking lots of water. It's much better if you drink fresh alkaline juices and purified water. You can take 1/2 ounce of alkaline every day to see positive results in your body weight.

4) The lungs are the organs that keep the blood purified. They allow oxygen to go directly into the bloodstream. It is also responsible for eliminating the waste gases found in every cell of the body. Deep breathing and fresh air are very useful to keep the lungs healthy and free of toxins. If you are in an urban area, it is recommended that you find an oxygen-rich area where you can take deep breaths.

5) The colon is the body's solid waste management organ. Doctors have found many people who may have up to 80 pounds of mucus and rubber-like solid waste found on the walls of the colon. Detoxifying and cleansing the colon can be a very difficult thing to do. However, having a waste-free colon can certainly provide you with the good benefits of having a clean, healthy body.

Regular exercise for walking

If you are experiencing some side signs/effects of detoxification, you can try regular walking exercise. Exercise is a good key to a healthy, fit body.

Drink plenty of lemon water

Many diet doctors also suggest that you drink plenty of lemon water. This is an effective way to maintain a very good circulation and can increase the rate of detoxification within the body.

Detoxification is an important factor for your beauty

Where is that wonderful product that could revive you?

How many times has your brain felt so slow that you can't even think clearly?

How many times have you felt so tired that even climbing a single flight of stairs costs you a lot?

Or what about those moments when you felt so "unpleasant" that even your best suit can't lift your spirits?

You've tried every known trick to keep you in shape and you've searched every shelf in the health and beauty aisle for that wonderful product that could revive you, but still hasn't done you any good.

Why don't you try looking at home and

in the product section of your grocery store?

What am I talking about? I'm talking detox.

Detox isn't just buckets of sweat on the gym floor, or starve to death!

It is a holistic approach to health and beauty. It ranges from diet and fitness to a sense of well-being. Try it for a weekend and start the new week with a renewed and more revived. Detoxifying your path to health and beauty is possible with a few things you might conveniently find in your home. With a sponge or a brush, scented candles, aromatic oils, herbal teas and a weekend off, "time for me", everything is ready to rejuvenate and renew.

A "Time for Me" weekend

It starts on a Friday:

Eat lightly (think salads and fruits).

Think salads and fruits!

Drink plenty of water throughout the day.

At night, dry slowly - sponge or brush with slow, long strokes. Move in one direction: up and toward your groin. Refresh yourself with tea or water, then immerse yourself in a bath of warm water and drops of aromatic bath oil. Light some scented candles while gradually adding cold water in half an hour, until your bath cools a little. This is the beginning of your new health and beauty routine. This process is done for the stimulation of blood vessels.

Dry yourself and dress warmly for bed.

It starts the next day:

Drink hot water with lemon. Take a walk while you take a deep breath. Take a steam bath or go swimming. You can also ask your partner or therapist to give you a massage. Once again, finish your health and beauty detox regimen with a dry massage brush and a bath.

Spend Sunday doing the whole process, but add another one

Activity

Make a list of people or things, such as your job, that are toxic to you. Evaluate how you should treat them to lessen their toxic effect. After this, pamper yourself or do meditation exercises. However, remember that you may experience excessive sweating, mild headaches, and rashes. These are signs that your body is releasing toxins and that they are temporary.

Detoxification is effective, safe, and cheap enough to be part of your weekly health and beauty routine. Just remember to avoid this during your period, pregnancy and illness.

Finally, talk to your doctor if you encounter any problems while detoxing.

How detoxification helps your overall health

Toxin levels are rising at alarming rates every day

Just consider the growing number of health problems (such as cancer, cardiovascular disease, obesity, headaches, fatigue, persistent cough, constipation, allergies, etc.) in today's world. Toxins exist both externally (outside our body) and internally (inside our body). Through food, toxins exist when there are chemicals, pesticides, food addictives or drugs. Through the environment, air and water pollution are the main areas of toxins. We get these external toxins when we eat, breathe or touch.

Internally, our bodies produce toxins as a normal daily function. For example, perspiring and cleaning our intestines are important elimination functions. A body decomposes when it cannot handle normal elimination processes well due to an overload of toxins. This is also when the body becomes susceptible to bacteria, yeasts and parasites that enter it.

The results are infections and diseases, and the body's inability to cope with them.

To help achieve better health, it is important, therefore, to detoxify and cleanse

How much you want to detox really depends on yourself and how "clean" you want your body to be. In fact, any simple change in your diet that prevents and eliminates the build-up of toxins is helpful. For example, drinking eight glasses of filtered water is easy to do every day.

Other dietary changes can also be made, such as eating more green leafy vegetables and foods rich in fiber. Lettuces are a green "wonder", full of nutrients. Eat lots of salads!

A more drastic measure of cleansing your body is to make complete fasting

Complete fasting helps give your body's organs a much-needed rest. In fact, Hippocrates (the "Father of Modern Medicine") believed that the body needs not only physical but also chemical rest. Chemical rest refers to the retention of food, thus giving the organs of the body the opportunity to discharge accumulated waste products and thus cleanse themselves.

However, before embarking on a serious detox or cleaning regimen, it is recommended that you seek professional advice. Excessive detoxification can also occur in some cases, when some people go to extremes and the body's essential nutrients are lost.

Are you feeling lazy?

Failure to find the underlying cause and

treatment can be a danger to your health.

I would venture to assume that the majority of the population feels a little slow on a regular basis. If you go through this condition for a long time, you may begin to feel that this has become a normal situation for you and you get used to it.

But not finding the underlying cause and treatment can be a danger to your health. If you feel slow, then it is a warning sign that something is not right, and an immediate investigation is in order, as to the cause. There may be many different reasons for this condition. Many of the things we do every day absolutely poison our system. If you are a smoker, you definitely need to detox. As you spend time with many or several detoxification programs, you may have reached a point where you can quit smoking more easily.

Here are some of the causes of slowness

1) Diet is of great importance. With all the pesticides and chemicals in our food today and nutrient deficient soil, it can be difficult to get the nutrients we need for a healthy life. It is possible to regain good health by changing your diet to organic foods that include eating more raw fruits and vegetables and fewer cooked foods and sugar products.

You may want to consider taking good supplements to get nutrients you wouldn't otherwise get. You can argue that organic foods are so expensive, but consider this; you can save a few dollars on cheaper packaged foods that may be loaded with preservatives, nitrates, etc., but what is the value of your health?

How long do you expect your body to function properly if you put degraded fuel on it? You've seen what it can do to a car. It's the same with your body. If you look closely at healthy-looking celebrities who are fit, they have a secret you don't have. Since their income depends on their personality and good looks, they are forced to give up the usual diets of the average American. They exercise, eat smaller portions and include many more raw foods, plus they drink a lot of water and this brings up the following topic.

2) *Dehydration!* Approximately 80% of Americans are semi-dehydrated and don't even know it. Without this precious liquid, our bodies (which are 2/3 of water) cannot function properly. Dehydration alone can cause laziness. If you are dehydrated, that means that the water level in your body is below normal for proper functioning. The management for this is to increase your fluid intake. The best thing is just pure water, about 8 cups a day. If drinking so much water seems too difficult, you can increase your water consumption with green or herbal teas.

These teas have a beneficial effect in that, as well as increasing water intake, they also provide antioxidants that help your immune system. So drink and feel better!

3) Through poor diet, lack of exercise, viruses, bacteria and parasites, digestive problems can occur. Here we have a whole series of problems to solve. If your body is toxic, then your liver and kidneys may be overloaded. You can handle a lot of this with a liver and kidney cleanse.

Dealing with parasites

Parasites can reside in any major organ of the body and cause more problems than slowness. Manage the parasite infestation first, possibly using an herbal solution found at your local health food store, followed by a kidney cleanse, and then a liver and colon cleanse. This is a course recommended by Dr. Hulda Clark. There's a lot of different cleanups you can do. To find the one that's right for you, go online and type in the liver or kidney cleanse and carefully check what's right for you.

4) Other forms of detoxification are

fasting and enemas.

   • Fasting is a centuries-old natural healing technique that works very well when done correctly.
   • Coffee or lemon enemas are excellent for cleaning the colon of old or impacted stool.
   • Certain herbs may also be useful for cleansing the colon, such as sacred peel (in moderation), aloe vera, flaxseed, and red raspberry.
   • Get plenty of fiber (with plenty of water). This helps keep you regular.
   • An overly toxic colon can eventually put impurities in your bloodstream and this will definitely make you feel lazy.

5) There has been much controversy over the years about the excess mercury in your teeth. A dentist once told me that if you look inside your mouth, the fillings you have may look smooth on the outside, but if you could look underneath the fillings it's a very different story. It looks very irregular and metals may be seeping into your system.

The mercury in the system is the most toxic non-radioactive metal in the body and about half of all silver fillings are mercury. A variety of health problems can occur, including brain, kidney, and lung damage, and has even been linked to autism. You can be tested for metal toxicity through a hair and urine analysis.

- If the test result is positive, you may want to consider removing them and replacing them with gold fillings.
- However, even after replacement, it can take months for the body to excrete these toxins.
- Research and find a dentist with an excellent reputation who has done replacement fillings. (For an

interesting fact, a friend told me that
his mother had had headaches for 20
years and that after all the fillings
were changed, she no longer had
headaches.

6) A relatively new technology has come
out to detoxify the body, and that is with
an ionic footbath. You put your feet in a
tub of warm water with a little sea salt.
Ionic footbaths work by sending a small
current that goes in a circuit through the
body and generates positively charged
ions.

The high concentration of the ion field
adheres to the negatively charged toxins,
neutralizing them, and the body is then
able to dispose of them through the
approximately 2000 pores found on the
soles of your feet. You will then be able to
experience the correct acidic-alkaline pH
balance as nature has proposed. It's
painless and takes about 30 minutes.

Water will change color according to the toxicity of the body, and also by the hardness or softness of the water, wherever it is found, geographically.

Watercolour indicators for detoxification of body organs

- Black or brown, liver.
- Orange; joints.
- Dark green; gallbladder.
- Yellowish green; the kidneys or urinary tract.
- White foam; lymph nodes draining.
- Red spots; blood clot material.
- Black spots; heavy metals.

In addition, independent studies have been conducted that show levels of mucus, heavy metals, and fat in the water after 30 minutes.

Help eliminate that feeling of

slowness and fatigue

As you can see, there are many things you can do to help eliminate that feeling of slowness and fatigue. But as always, consult your doctor before doing any detoxification program.

Different types of detoxification cleanings

Regimens Your body should be cleansed naturally, but today's diets make the process difficult

Many resort to internal body cleansing to remove waste products and toxins. A detoxification treatment is designed to help the body eliminate stored toxins and strengthen the organs involved in this process.

Colon Cleanse

Colon cleansing helps cleanse the organ that assists the body in removing waste. A dirty colon can lead to a buildup of toxins in the body and disease. Through the use of herbal treatments or irrigation therapy, a cleansing of the colon removes toxins and helps the intestinal tract function properly. It is essential to do this cleaning first, so that residues produced by other detoxification procedures can be efficiently disposed of.

Cleaning the kidneys

His kidneys clean about 200 pints of blood daily. A kidney cleanse will help your kidneys function more efficiently. It usually involves consuming a large amount of water or juice and then eliminating everything to remove the kidneys.

Liver Cleanse

Your liver completes about two dozen processes for the body daily, and cleansing this important organ helps the liver support the immune system and support the digestive functions of the body. There are several supplements and liver purge programs available.

Pulmonary Cleaning

Cleaning the lungs is also important for

good health. American diets high in dairy products often produce lung fatty tissue. Cleaning the lungs alleviates this problem.

Skin cleansing

Finally, cleansing the skin releases toxins lodged in the fat layers just beneath the skin. Most are made with herbs, saunas and sweat lodges.

"Clean" and Running Smoothly

Cleaning your body of toxins is a great way to keep your systems "clean" and running smoothly. The results are worth it:

Improves the immune system

Lighter skin complexion

Sleep better

Acne Cure

Cure of constipation

Disappearance of unpleasant body odours

... Just to name a few! In short, you will be surprised at the conditions that will be clarified!

Here are some ideas for a detox diet.

There are several types of detox diets

There are some where you can only eat fruits and vegetables. Those where you can only eat "clean" foods and those where you can only drink fruit and vegetable juice and even the most extreme where you can only drink water.

You can also do specialized cleanings designed specifically for certain areas of the body, such as the liver, kidneys, blood, or lungs. However, most detox diets only involve cleansing the entire body.

A sample of a seven-day detox diet you can try

First, it is important that you have regular bowel movements during a detox because this will decrease the likelihood that the toxins will be reabsorbed by the body. A good way to make sure you eliminate regularly is to take 2 tablespoons of flax seeds ground in lemon water in the morning and drink lemon water throughout the day. Linseed provides the body with fibre and lemon water has a slightly laxative effect.

It is also important to drink enough fluids in a cleanse. You should try to include at least 8 glasses of water a day to make sure you are allowing the toxins to be eliminated.

A sample menu of a detox diet.

This is a diet that allows for some food as it tends to be easier for beginners.

Remember, you can modify this to suit your needs and preferences.

IN RETURN

1/2 lemon squeezed in a glass of warm water

1 tablespoon of bentonite clay and 1 tablespoon of ground flax seeds in a glass of water

BREAKFAST

Breakfast shake based on pear, rice milk and rice protein powder

Supplements: Vitamin C

MOCADILLOS

Apple juice diluted with water

Water

Vegetable broth

Supplements: milk thistle

Celery and hummus sticks

LUNCH

Vegetable soup with chunks made with vegetable broth and your choice of vegetables

Steamed broccoli with sesame seeds and beets sprinkled with lemon juice over brown rice

Apple sauce

Supplements: Multivitamin

MOCADILLOS

Dandelion Root Tea

Carrot sticks with hummus sauce

Water

Supplements: Milk Thistle

DINNER

Lentils with curry on quinoa

Salad with mixed vegetables, red peppers, artichokes and sprouts drizzled with garlic salad dressing, lemon juice and olive oil.

Vegetable broth

BEFORE GOING TO BED

1 tablespoon of bentonite clay and 1 tablespoon of ground flax seeds in a glass

of water

This can be followed for up to seven days.

Relax and enjoy your cleaning time, and remember to be careful, because although you should expect to feel slow and slightly sick, if you feel very sick or fatigued, contact your doctor.

An Additional Plan

A Detox Diet Plan Is Not Targeted at Weight Loss

Its goal is to cleanse and revitalize the body by combining natural organic foods, herbs and simple exercises to purge the body of accumulated toxins. Over time, consumption of processed foods, non-vegetarian foods, and sugars leads to clogging of the inner walls of the colon with debris.

This results in an overload of internal cleansing organs such as the liver and kidneys. They become slow, allowing toxins and bacteria to re-enter the circulatory system instead of being completely eliminated through feces, urine, or sweat.

These toxins produce fatigue, infections of the skin and other organs, migraines, flatulence, heartburn, constipation and many other serious diseases. A regular diet detoxification plan can rid the body of accumulated toxins and lead to an active, disease-free life. Detoxification is not appropriate for children! However, an excellent diet filled with natural foods found in a detox diet, ARE very appropriate!

1 Day Detox Plan

This diet is not for diabetics, patients with low blood pressure, anorexics or teenagers, as it does not provide enough fuel for their physical activities. It can be a one-week diet of raw organic liquids, fruits and vegetables to clean the system.

Gradually reintroduce other foods, but refrain from non-vegetarian and processed foods. Certain natural herbs can also be used. This is a simple and quick way to revitalize your system, after a binge or an excess of indulgence.

TOMORROW

➢ A glass of pomegranate juice (the most powerful natural antioxidant).

➢ Some almonds (source of oil and proteins).

➢ Mid-morning snack

➢ A bowl of brown rice (a source of vitamins and minerals in carbohydrates).

➢ A little tofu (protein).

➢ Lunch

➢ A glass of pomegranate juice.

➢ A large portion of mixed green salad (provides essential nutrients and bulk) sprinkled with a teaspoon of olive oil or vinegar.

➢ Midday snack

➢ A glass of pomegranate juice.

➢ A handful of almonds.

➢ Dinner

➢ A glass of pomegranate juice.

➢ A big bowl of brown rice.

➢ Drink at least 8-10 glasses of water a day.

This detox diet will provide you with 1200 calories and healthy nutrition to remove toxins from your body in 24 hours. It can help you lose about 600 grams of body weight and, if followed regularly once a week, will keep your body healthy and active.

Detoxify your body and build a strong, healthy immune system

A natural process through which your body passes

Detoxification is a natural process that your body goes through and removes wastes known as toxins. Under normal conditions, our bodies are designed to eliminate these toxins through the liver, kidneys, lymphatic system, skin, etc.

There are many reasons why detoxification is so important

In these times there is the problem of our chemical environment due to air and water pollutants. There is also the fact that most of our food is grown with pesticides in an effort to reduce insect and bacterial infestation in order to produce higher yields. All you need to do is go to the supermarket and read the labels to see how many colorants and preservatives you eat every day.

Step back in time

If you had to take a step back in time (even only 30 to 40 years), you would realize how different we ate then. If you didn't grow your own organic food, you would probably have gone to your butcher daily and bought fresh, hormone-free meat, and then gone to the market to buy fresh, organic produce.

The word "organic" probably wasn't something that would have been associated with food back then. You would have associated the word with a biology class.

Today we are severely lacking in

nutrients

The air we breathe constantly is a little polluted. We drink high fructose drinks, eat lots of preserves and consume an incredible amount of sodium. I'm not saying we never eat this way, because we all like to indulge from time to time, but if we eat a normal American diet high in salt, sugar and preservatives, and canned goods, then we may be doing ourselves a disservice. It may feel full, but it lacks many nutrients.

There are several things you can do to undo the toxicity

It is almost impossible to be completely free of all pollutants in our environment, but anything you can do to relieve your body from the accumulation of toxins and malnutrition should be beneficial to your health.

Hot baths or Sauna

Liver and kidney cleanings are excellent,

but if you're not inclined to do this, then there are other solutions... like taking a hot bath for half an hour, or sweating toxins in a sauna.

Clean

If you feel compelled to do these cleanings, then make sure you have eaten well and drank up to 8 glasses of water, so that your blood sugar level does not drop and so that you stay well hydrated during the process. Not only does it lose toxins this way, but it also loses water, salt, and potassium, which can make you feel dizzy.

Herbal teas

There are some great herbal teas that you can drink on a regular basis that also gently cleanse the body, moisturize, have antioxidant properties, and help eliminate toxins. It's a warm and refreshing way to relax and do good to the body.

Fruit and Vegetable Juice

Fruit and vegetable juice is a fantastic way to get more nutrients into the body, because you are maintaining the integrity of the nutrients. If you are putting the vegetables in a boiling pot, then you will have nutrient loss. This is called bleaching and all the goodness enters the water. If you overcook the food and then flush the water, then your nutrients just went down the drain, and you're ingesting the rest of the whitened shell.

Raw or with juice is the way to go!

It is advisable to take supplements that strengthen your immune system.

Because we have a nutrient deficient soil, it is advisable to take supplements that strengthen your immune system, such as Q-10, and vitamins A, D, E, C and B. Trace elements and electrolytes are necessary to keep our systems in shape. Avoid high-sugar sports drinks, but instead get good-quality electrolytes at a health food store.

If nothing else, then at least get a good multivitamin to take every day.

You got a headache? Are you tired?

Are you overweight or tired all the time? Do you have headaches, other aches and pains, frequent colds and flu, constipation or digestive problems, high blood pressure, premenstrual syndrome, allergies or sensitivities? Do you often drink too much alcohol, drink caffeinated beverages, smoke cigarettes, use over-the-counter or recreational drugs, or eat fast, fried or refined foods?

Detoxification for Rescue

Our bodies have a natural detoxification system (composed of the digestive tract, urinary system and liver) that helps process all the chemicals that modern life throws at you. These chemicals are called "toxins", they are basically poisons that have harmful effects on the body. Not only alcohol and tobacco are loaded with toxins; pesticides and food additives, caffeine and pollution also play an important role.

Benefits of a Detox Diet

Detox diets are believed to prevent chronic diseases, such as arthritis, heart disease, and cancer.

2. People who try a detox diet often find that it can improve toxicity symptoms such as fatigue, joint pain, headache, pain, premenstrual syndrome, unhealthy skin, poor concentration, anxiety and irritability, frequent colds, heartburn, constipation, and gas.

3. Detox diets may be recommended as part of a supervised treatment plan for chronic diseases such as autoimmune diseases, multiple chemical sensitivities, fibromyalgia, chronic fatigue syndrome, digestive disorders, heart disease, and arthritis.

Detoxification Tips

➢ Clear your daily detox period from any pub, club, restaurant or party. See it as an opportunity to do all those things you never get to, like visiting museums and galleries - then you can feel doubly satisfied in the end when you're not only healthier, but also more educated.

➢ Drink plenty of water to avoid dehydration.

➢ Take milk thistle to optimize these benefits; it contains silymarin, which protects the liver from damage.

Detoxification of mind and body:

Special chiropractic treatments for drug addicts have been shown to be very successful in stabilizing those who withdraw from drugs and other addictive behaviors.

Mind-Body Detox is being recognized by scientific and medical professionals and their publications around the world. Chiropractors who use activating methods to treat ill health, pain and even addiction are sought out by addicts who wish to overcome their addiction. The mind-body detoxification process gently activates movement - without bursting the bones - which stimulates the brain's pleasure receptors and positively affects emotions.

Juice Fasting

Are you stressed from the overload?

Because of the highly processed foods we eat and the polluted air we breathe, our bodies accumulate toxins. The body does everything possible to eliminate toxins, but ends up stressed because of the overload. Symptoms such as chronic headaches, skin allergies, premature aging, etc. begin to manifest themselves.

What can we do to help our sick body? Try juice fasting as a safe way to detox!

Many studies have been conducted on the beneficial effects of juice fasting. We can increase our life expectancy, treat biochemical imbalances, reduce our cholesterol levels, treat allergies, acne, etc.

In juice fasting, by giving the body a break from food and digestion, the immune system can focus on the elimination of toxins, with the help of elimination organs (liver, pancreas, gallbladder, kidneys, intestines, skin, etc.).

A prolonged fast (3 more days)

During a prolonged fast (more than 3 days), the body will begin to burn and digest its own tissues, by autolysis process, in a discriminated way. It first breaks down and burns those cells and tissues that are diseased, damaged, aged or dead (tumors, morbid cells, abscesses, excess fat, etc.). The stomach shrinks and becomes less acidic.

Then, certain detoxification symptoms are experienced, for example, acne breakouts, fatigue, headaches, as the body eliminates its toxins. These symptoms should be relieved and we will feel a renewed sense of health and well-being!

You can juice almost any fruit and vegetable you can eat raw.

Vegetables that are good for juicing include tomatoes, cucumbers, celery, and carrots.

Combinations of fruits and vegetables taste delicious

For example, apple and carrot juice makes a good mix. Another good combination is apple, celery and tomato.

In the case of fruit and vegetable peels, peel them, especially if you suspect they have been sprayed. If you can use organic fruit, this will be much better. Rinse with filtered or distilled water.

How to Make Juice?

It is recommended to dilute your juice 50/50 with water, especially if you are using fruits and the juice is too sweet. Use distilled water, if possible, for dilution.

The juice has to be prepared fresh!

Remember, you can't buy freshly made juice from a grocery store or any juice from a package, despite what the package label says. Any juice in a cardboard box, can or bottle has been heat treated for preservation. The juice must be prepared fresh! The longer the juice stays out, the fewer raw and fresh food enzymes it will contain. This means you can find a store that prepares it just before you drink it, or you can use a juicer yourself.

8 benefits for juice fasting

There are many benefits to juices, especially if you prepare them yourself:

8 benefits of juice fasting

1. If drunk fresh, the juice is full of live enzymes, which helps the body.

2. Unlike coming out of a package, the juice is fresh and not pasteurized. Pasteurization has its advantages, but has resulted in nutritionally dead foods. During pasteurization, high heat is used and this destroys vital nutrients within the juice.

3. You eat more vegetables when you drink than when you eat. As you have probably experienced, it is not always possible to eat as many vegetables as you would like. Drinking fresh vegetable juice helps solve this problem.

4. Digestion and assimilation of plant

nutrients is much easier. Your body is, in fact, like a squeezer. When you eat celery, your body digests it by extracting the juice for nutrition. Fiber is eliminated through the colon and stool. However, if you juice, you have already extracted the juice for the body, which facilitates its assimilation. However, it is still important to eat whole vegetables and fruits, because a certain amount of fiber is also needed.

5. Fasting rests your digestive system. Because fresh fruit and vegetable juices require little digestion, they assimilate quickly into your body. Most of the 10% of the body's energy normally involved in its assimilation, digestion and elimination is released. The end result? You feel a sense of renewed energy after fasting.

6. Fasting also helps break down toxic materials - fats, abnormal cells, and tumors - and releases diseased tissues and their cellular products into the circulation for elimination.

7. In addition, the growth of new cells during fasting is stimulated and accelerated as the required proteins are re-synthesized from broken down cells (during autolysis). The reading of serum albumin, that is, the level of protein in the blood, remains constant and normal throughout your fast, as your body uses very intelligently the proteins and other nutrients stored when needed.

8. Juice fasting is a much milder detoxification process compared to fasting in water. For a juice fast, a wide variety of fruits and vegetables should be used in combination, as this is necessary to improve health during fasting. In this way, the body still gets its daily calories from easily digested juices compared to the faster extreme water. Therefore, the release of toxins from fat cells in a juice fast is milder and gradual.

Incredible juice recipes for fasting

All you need is a juicer!

Juice fasting is gaining popularity as a great way to detoxify. Many people are interested in removing toxins from their bodies in order to lead healthier lives. When toxins build up in the body, they feel slow and also have a deficient immune system. Juice fasting, as a cleansing method, can help people achieve better health and more energy.

It is very easy to do as the fruits are easy to obtain and all that is required in addition is a juicer.

If you are a beginner

For a beginner to juice fasting, it is important to start slowly and try it for a day. By fasting on juice, you are limiting your consumption to juices only. Fruit juices are high in sugar, so if you are diabetic or need to control your sugar intake, you should be careful when trying to fast with fruit juices. Anyone who is starting to fast should always talk to their doctor first. Also, do not drink juice on an empty stomach for long periods of time, such as more than 3 days, unless your doctor agrees that it is safe for you to do so.

The following pages are examples of recipes that can help you get an idea of fruit and vegetable combinations to use together.

Recipe 1: *Vegetable Juice Combo*

Vegetable Juice Combo

2 sheets of chard

1/2 beetroot

2 or 3 sprigs of watercress

3 carrots

1 stalk celery

Wash with filtered or distilled water; cut and place in blender.

Recipe 2: *Carrot and apple juice*

Carrot and apple juice

2-3 Green Apples

1 carrot

Fresh basil leaves

Wash with filtered or distilled water; cut and place in blender.

Recipe 3: *Carrot - Vegetable Juice*

Carrot - Vegetable Juice

A handful of dandelion leaves

1 leaf kale

4 carrots

Leaves of fresh mint, basil or cilantro

Wash with filtered or distilled water; cut and place in blender.

Recipe 4: Peach Juice

Peach Juice

2 or 3 peaches

Wash with filtered or distilled water; cut and place in blender.

There are many different types of juice fasting. Some diets require fruit juices, while others use fewer sugary vegetable juices. You can always come up with your own unique combination of diet recipes for fruit and vegetable juices!

How to prevent cancer through a detox diet?

Cancer is very common today

It may be a loved one, a relative, or your next-door neighbor who has cancer and is now desperately trying to find a cure for the cancer. Finding a cure when you are already diagnosed with cancer is definitely more difficult and heartbreaking than adopting good cancer prevention habits in the first place. Learning to prevent cancer is a necessity for everyone because cancer does not discriminate, anyone can get it.

To treat and prevent cancer, new ideas are being launched every day.

But all of them are based on a healthy lifestyle. Following a detox diet is a new form of cancer prevention that has really taken off.

Preventing cancer is possible if you keep your body healthy and free of toxins.

Eating healthy is always advisable, no matter what disease you are struggling with. The reason for this is that healthy foods contain vitamins and have properties that make your body work better. A body that functions properly and at an efficient level stays healthier.

Exercise

That brings us to exercise. Exercise helps your body burn fat and keeps your muscles toned. It also helps the heart and lungs function better, allowing blood to flow better and keeping waste moving through the body properly. Maintaining a healthy lifestyle prepares your body to be healthy.

A detox diet

A detox diet helps your body's organs work at their optimal level and without blockages. Helps eliminate toxins from the body and eliminate waste more efficiently. A detox program usually involves a lot of fiber and water, and gives your body's organs a rest. Fiber helps your body eliminate waste, freeing your system to better digest food.

This, in turn, gives you more energy. Water has an overall effect on your energy levels and the functioning of your body. Instead of letting wastes build up and cause many problems, the detox diet removes wastes from your body and releases your colon. Simply put, the detox diet allows your colon to return to work and your colon to function optimally once again. A colon that isn't working can only result in cancer.

Not all causes of cancer are known, but taking the time to be healthier in cancer prevention can do a lot for your health and your future.

What are the side effects of detoxification?

Our bodies are able to detoxify chemicals on their own.

However, many experts believe that the enormous number of chemicals we ingest daily through food, water and the environment can accumulate.

Toxic Cargo or Body Cargo

Accumulation, called toxic load or body burden, can overwhelm the body's ability to detoxify and can lead to hormonal imbalance, nutritional deficiency, and inefficient metabolism.

What are the possible side effects of a detox diet?

Some people may experience headache, acne, weight loss, or fatigue during detoxification. These symptoms usually subside after a few days. For this reason, many people take time off from work to start a detox or diet on a Friday night.

Replace your biggest vices with healthier alternatives

Remember that your organs will benefit

from any kind of rest, so you can always opt for an intermediate option where you replace your larger vices with healthier alternatives.

Side effects of detoxification

1. Many people experience headaches at the beginning of a detox as their bodies adapt to the dramatic reduction of their daily poisons. That's why it's worth cutting the main vices slowly before you start;

2. Your energy may decrease before you get up, so it's worth starting the program one weekend for your body to adjust. Drink Caffeinated Beverages? Most Americans do. And with the stress of our society, it's hard not to. Even if you're not ready to quit smoking forever, a spring and fall detox can give your liver a chance to rest from detoxifying all that caffeine every day, and that can have tremendous physical benefits in terms of more energy, better sleep, and reduced stress.... which, in turn, can also make it possible to significantly reduce caffeine after your detox.

Fresh fruit

Enjoy all the fresh fruit. Again... Careful with the grapefruit! A compound in grapefruit called naringin can significantly inhibit liver detoxification enzymes and should be avoided during detoxification diets.

Conclusion: Economic Health

Serious socio-economic problems?

Can you tell me what is the most common problem facing young Americans today?

Well, most of you will fill your brains with serious socio-economic problems, while in reality it is the degenerate health of the current generation that has become a cause for concern, not only among medical authorities, but also among social scientists. The similarities are terrifying.

Degeneration of health in the U.S.

You may be wondering why it bothers social scientists, because the deterioration in the overall health of average Americans is directly related to their accelerated lifestyle. Grabbing hamburgers while running and washing them with bottles of soda - what a sad syndrome! And it has become synonymous with our national characteristics.

The harmful effects of surviving on junk food

Just try to remember how many obese people you face every day on your way to work, and you'll see for yourself the harmful effects of surviving on junk food. Excessive weight gain, lethargy, constipation... names them and includes them all on the list of impacts that junk food has on our health and our lives.

We're all human, and sometimes we just crave a meal like this. We've almost been culturally trained to eat this way! As you retrain your habits, I can almost guarantee that these cravings will go away. One of the main reasons many people eat this way is for convenience, and we all lead such busy lives. Inspect your priorities!

Overflowing with junk food and a dietary habit that is low in fiber and moisture actually fills our internal system with toxins and when the colon becomes clogged with impacted fecal matter for years, the toxins cannot be removed from our system, adding more injuries to our health that manifest in these physical and mental disorders.

The Importance of Colon Detoxification

Now you can understand the importance of colon detoxification. Detoxification is a process to remove toxins first from the colon and then from the entire body, or neutralize or transform them.

Impacted waste from the colon is expelled from the body in the process. Colon detoxification means cleansing the colon to remove hardened layers of mucoid plaques from the colon. Any program of detoxification of our body begins with the cleansing of the colon and that is not without reason.

The colon is the last point in our body's food processing system. Therefore, if this organ remains full of waste, any attempt to detoxify other organs such as the kidney or liver will be in vain, as the toxins generated there will be recycled back into your system. And then your system will be threatened by even more serious complications... such as cancer or the failure of the immune system.

However, don't be frightened because you feel that your colon is not in its proper state of good health! There's actually a great deal you can do to change it for the better. Several proven methods throughout the time of colon detoxification can help you return to your previous state of health and help you... Enjoy life to the fullest.

Regular colon cleanse

Enema, herbal supplement, oxygen-based colon cleansers, colon irrigation....

you can benefit from a number of sophisticated colon cleansing techniques. Remember, your body's detoxification program begins in your colon and regular colon cleansing ensures overall well-being.

Fast food and milk shakes

Therefore, the next time you gorge yourself on a young man gorging himself on fast food and milkshakes (yes, even if YOU are the culprit and have given him all these "treats"), inform him about their harmful effects, as well as the advantages of colon detoxification to get rid of the damage he has already done to his system. Children and young people who grow up knowing the health facts about food are much more likely to take care of their bodies even when they are away from home, away from their help and instruction, and making decisions in a world pressured by their peers.

Just remember that everything will not

happen overnight and that it will take time before you see a change in your life for the better.

Now yes, I wish you the best in your results, and remember, everything is practical; theory without action is of no use to you. It brings everything you learn into real life.

A big hug, your friend, Jessy!

By the way, when you achieve your results little by little, I highly recommend you, if you want to learn much more about methods of detoxification, I highly recommend you, the book of a great friend of mine, on "RED TEA DEINTOXICATION TO LOSE WEIGHT", is a book that I am sure will help you a lot on your way to "good health". Without further ado, you can find it in the search engine of Amazon, as: "Detoxification of red tea to lose weight" or looking for its name, as: "Agustin R. Ruiz"... Once again I wish you success in your results!